# How to Beat Anxiety and

# Panic Attacks!

**A Registered Nurse's Way to Put Anxiety
and Panic Attacks to an End**

# HOW TO BEAT ANXIETY AND PANIC ATTACKS!

## A REGISTERED NURSE'S WAY TO PUT ANXIETY AND PANIC ATTACKS TO AN END

Written by T.L. CAMPBELL, M.S.N., R.N.

**COMING TO AUDIBLE.COM**

**Late 2018**

**NOTICE:**

If you are finding yourself in a situation where you are having homicidal or suicidal thoughts or ideations, or if you feel you are having an emergency then you should **CALL 911 NOW!**

✳ ✳ ✳

Dear Reader,

My name is Trace Campbell, M.S.N., R.N. and I have been a practicing nurse for 10 years. I hold a Master of Science Degree in Nursing, Management and Leadership. I am currently the Vice President of Clinical and Business Operations for Nav-Central in Texas, and currently working to completing my Doctorate.

In my many years of working with mixed-populations in the healthcare arena I have encountered my fair share of anxiety, panic attacks, and other psychological disorders in my patients, and in myself.

For 10 years I suffered from anxiety disorder and panic attacks. I'm happy to say that those days are now in the distant past.

There were a lot of different situations that initially brought me to the point where I was spiraling out of control.

I was working a dead-end job as a retail manager for Office Max, struggling to make ends meet. I would pray every night, and for years, for God to help me with the disabling anxiety I was experiencing, and to put me in a place where I could handle the oppressive disorder and the beat down of the nightly panic attacks.

For years, I wasn't even aware what it was that I was actually experiencing. *Why was I so nervous about certain situations that arose in my life? Why wouldn't I leave my home, to go places, to see friends, or visit family on holidays, or for special occasions? Why would I wake from sleep in sheer panic?*

I didn't know the answer. I didn't know what the problem was, or even that I had a problem at all. I thought it was just normal stress, and that I was just handling it poorly.

All I knew was that no matter what I did, everything seemed dark and hopeless. I was always worried, and stressed, and afraid, and exhausted.

No matter where I turned or what I did to stop feeling so badly, a dark cloud of impending doom hung above me, following my every move, threatening to unleash a torrent of never-ending and drowning oppression on me and my life. My very sanity seemed to be in danger.

At first, the feelings of anxiety came and went pretty quickly, poking and prodding at the edges of my mind, looking for a way inside me. But as time went on, there were more episodes, and they came more frequently and subsided slower as anxiety found an entrance and began to latch on.

After about a year, I found that I would wake from a troubled sleep; my chest would be tight, I would become short of breath. I would be covered in a cold sweat, and I was scared of some *'thing'* that was unknown to me.

This led to sleep disorders because I was afraid of going to sleep and waking up with a panic attack.

After a while of letting the anxiety and panic attacks have their way with me, the situation began to really get out hand.

The thing is, if you let your problems take root and grow within you, they go from being acute and happening all of the sudden, to being a chronic condition and always being present in your life. Your mind and body become accustomed to registering the unknown fear and reacting in a certain way because it seems an appropriate response to the invisible threat.

As a registered nurse I understand that there are two types of stress. One is beneficial and helps us stay sharp, observant, and presses us to be better at meeting the challenges that daily life presents. It keeps us safe in dangerous situations.

The second, is an anxiety that just takes control of us and ragdolls us across the living room, at its every whim, where we just land in a nervous heap in the corner and concede that anxiety is the victor.

I finally got the point in my life where I was tired of dealing with the beating that this problem was causing me. I still didn't know what was going on. I thought that maybe I had become ill with some horrible disease.

I started calling and making doctor's appointments. I would go and get seen in the clinics, but not one doctor could tell me what was causing the symptoms I was experiencing. Almost continuously at this point.

I called the nurse hotlines so much that after a while they got to know me on a first name basis. After a while they had told me all they could. I was a frequent flyer, and though I was always friendly they were unable to help me. They would advise me that they were sorry, but I needed to see my provider for further evaluation. The circle was complete. I was back to where I started, and the problem was only getting worse.

I started to really focus on attacks and realized there was a connection with daily stress and the timing of some of the events. I drew the conclusion that I was suffering, not from a physical condition, but rather from a psychological disorder, and I said, ENOUGH!

In time I was able to get control of the situation and take my life back. I want to help you transform your life too. I know that together we can help you beat anxiety and panic. Exactly the same way I beat it.

I help thousands of people every year take control of their lives and I have full confidence and faith that I can help you too.

Let's start by writing this day down on a calendar. Mark it as the first day you decided to take back control over your own life.

Together we will learn the steps that will help you make the changes to your life that will release you of the throat-clenching prison you have been chained within up until now.

You may want to know how this book differs from any other on the market today?

It's simple really, because most books focus on treating the symptoms that anxiety causes, thereby creating a reoccurring anxiety and panic for the patient; a continuous never-ending cycle of fear. Those books do not address the main cause of the problem. They only treat the symptoms.

*How to Beat Anxiety and Panic Attacks! A Registered Nurse's Way to Put Anxiety and Panic Attacks to an End*, focuses on the Root Cause of the problem. It teaches you how to turn it off at the source, and retrain your brain, so that it doesn't come back... ever again!

I don't know everything there is to know about anxiety, but I know how it abused me for years, and I know how my patients feel when they call me for help.

People who call me are on the edge. They are begging for help. They may even be ready to end it all.

I have dealt with everything from a little chest tightness to full-blown suicidal situations, and every single time I have been able to help myself, and my patients.

You may think you're different because you have this problem, and you may think you are alone, with no chance of getting help, but I am here to tell you that you are not alone. You are not different. You can make this problem disappear for good. THERE IS A CURE FOR ANXIETY!

Anxiety disorders are a tangled maze of thought processes, chemical hormones, actions, emotions, and a lack of understanding for what is happening, what is causing it, or how to make it go away for good. When you are deep inside the maze it's hard to see the way out over the tops of the hedges, but just like with any maze, there *is* a way out. You only have to find it.

I am a testament to the fact that this disorder can be beaten. My patients are living proof that you can be victorious over anxiety and not let it control your every move or thought.

When I began writing this book, and its companion, 30 Day Workbook and Therapeutic Journal, I asked myself, what do people need to know about anxiety and panic attacks, and how can I write this book so that it can actually helps someone understand how to beat it? I decided it's best to break the book into 3 parts.

In Part I we will take a look at the many-headed beast that is '*anxiety*' and the forms it takes, and what causes each to be triggered. We will determine how, exactly, you are supposed to address them when they occur.

In Part II you will learn how to fight anxiety and put a choke hold on panic attacks. Remember you are stronger than panic. You are stronger than fear. You are stronger than anxiety. You will soon have the tools you need to go into battle and slay your dragon.

Part III will take everything we have discussed and put it all together for you, so you can continue to win and cure yourself of the anxiety you are feeling and panic attacks you are experiencing.

The goal of this book is not to make you feel better, which it will, but its true purpose is about long-term and lasting results and improving your outcome to deal with this situation once and for all.

It's important that you don't skip anything in this book, no matter how badly you want to get to the end. Consume each part of this book. Learn it well, understand it thoroughly, and live it every day.

I strongly encourage you to go to Amazon.com and purchase the paperback, *HOW TO BEAT ANXIETY AND PANIC ATTACKS! A Registered Nurse's Way to Put Anxiety and Panic Attacks to an End: **The 30-Day Workbook and Therapeutic Journal***, by T.L. Campbell. It was written specially to retrain your mind and get on track to controlling your anxiety and panic attacks.

*Now... Let's Get Better!*

# Part I: A Registered Nurse's Way to Put Anxiety and Panic Attacks to and End!

Let me introduce you to Lee, Dawn, and Rose.

**LEE** is a 28-year-old retail manager who had recently become separated from his wife of 10 years.

It was the first time Lee had been alone, as he had gone from graduating and living at home with his parents to living with his spouse.

The only place Lee could find to live was a run-down apartment in the city, which was a far cry from the home in the gated community he had shared with his wife. He was accustomed to the laid back, peaceful environment that the community had offered.

Now he was living in a crime ridden area in the middle of the city. He was surrounded by the sound of cars, and loud car stereos, and loud-talking people coming and going at all hours of the day and night.

Either from the stress of the divorce , or the constant noise of the big city apartment complex to which he was unaccustomed, Lee started to have problems sleeping.

The job he had held as a manager for the past 5 years began to suffer due to the stress of the divorce combined with a lack of sleep.

His boss began to notice and called Lee in to talk about his dip in performance. Lee now began to worry that his job might be in danger, and if he lost his job, he'd lose his apartment and might even become homeless.

This situation escalated, and though Lee didn't lose his job he began waking in fear several times per night. His chest was tight, and he had to pant to catch his breath. He was sweating profusely and was unable to fall back to sleep.

As the weeks went by these episodes became more and more common for Lee, and things became worse. He was worried all the time now and no matter what he tried he couldn't stop worrying. Soon he found he was worried about everything and turned to alcohol to relax.

The alcohol made the sleeping problems worse, Lee was tired all the time. He was worried he was going to lose his job. He was worried he would be alone and homeless for the rest of his life. Lee had gone from an acute phase of anxiety to a chronic phase in just a few short months.

**DAWN**, a 34-year-old single mother of 2 felt that she wasn't loved by her children and that she had no friends to talk to about her life.

Her boyfriend is out of work, and she only works part time, which isn't enough to make ends meet. To make matters worse her 14-year-old daughter has become pregnant.

She didn't feel she could cope and that everything was spinning out of control in her life. As time went by she became withdrawn and made excuses to miss family events.

It became so bad, in fact, that the anxiety manifested itself in physical ways with nausea, shortness of breath, and diarrhea. She began to fear that she was becoming ill, that she was dying of some horrible disease. I know exactly how she felt.

The doctors could find nothing physically wrong with her. Depression was setting in and in time she wouldn't leave the safety of her room or talk to anyone. As her anxiety progressed she began to foster thoughts of self-harm.

**ROSE**, a 71-year-old widow living alone with no support group of family or friends.

She doesn't know where to turn. She feels like her life is over since her husband died. Her bills began to pile up and her limited income wasn't enough to catch up. Th bill collectors began to hound her night and day.

She found herself pacing the floor at all hours of the night. Even though she realized she was anxious, she didn't know how to help herself. She had begun to accept that she was alone, and life would be miserable from that point forward.

These three people were burdened by the strain of everyday life, and they lost the ability to cope with the stress of events. In time each developed anxiety disorder and panic attacks.

After years of fighting, what for them seemed to be a losing battle, they each confided in me. They are now committed to mastering the techniques provided within this book and the companion workbook and journal. They are living happier lives with fewer bouts of anxiety and are now prepared to recognize the signs of anxiety and have all the tools to fight and win against anxiety and panic attacks.

## The Negative Voice

It is very important to stay positive, think the positive, and speak the positive. If you start thinking that Lee, Dawn, and Rose were any different than you, and that the techniques in this book won't help you the same way, then you'd be wrong. That's just negative thinking.

If you say "Well, I just can't do this, it will never work for me because my situation is different," that's negative speaking, and it will be a downfall for you every time. That's why you must read this book, every page, from front to back, and refer to it as often as you need to.

Please, don't think that just because your situation is different from Lee's, Dawn's, and Rose's, that you can't be helped. These are just three people out of the millions who share the disorder of anxiety.

## What is Anxiety?

People all over this big, beautiful, blue planet we call Earth experience many different levels of stress every day. Anxiety is a normal reaction to stressful situations. There all kinds of stressful situations for instance: taking an exam, problems with a child or spouse, visiting a doctor's office or dentist, the noisy neighbor next door that loves to play his radio, very loudly, at 2 o'clock in the morning.

There are multiple types of anxiety disorders, and people who have an anxiety disorder have a difficult time coping with the situation when it occurs.

Disorders dealing with anxiety are a form of mental illness, and people who have this particular disorder have differing levels reaction to triggering events. In some cases, an episode of anxiety can keep us from carrying out activities of their daily lives.

People who have such a disorder constantly worry about things that are happening in their lives. They can become fearful, paranoid, confused, lose focus, and completely become disabled by the level of anxiety they are experiencing.

The term Anxiety Disorder is an umbrella term, which includes many different conditions.

Some of the signs and symptoms of anxiety are:

**Dizziness**

**Nausea**

Heart Palpitations

Cold, tingling, sweaty, and/or numb
hands and feet.

Sleep problems (insomnia)

Panic attacks

Feelings of hopelessness

Feelings of impending doom

Chest tightness

Dry mouth

Muscle tension

Shortness of breath

**Inability to calm**

**Inability to remain still (pacing, fidgeting)**

Providers, scientists, and researchers have been looking for the cause of anxiety for year, but the truth is, that no one really knows what causes this disorder.

Much like any other physical or mental illness the cause of problem may come from chemical or structural changes in your brain, environmental factors, social stress and genetics, to name a few, and can affect the parts of your brain that help with coping, handling fear and paranoia, and other emotions that when triggered could set off a chain link of events for anxiety to present itself.

As a Registered Nurse if you have any of the signs or symptoms listed above, I strongly encourage you to see your healthcare provider immediately to be evaluated.

Some of these signs and symptoms could be urgent or even life threatening, and serious situations should be ruled out by a doctor.

If you experience any of these signs or symptoms and can not speak to a nurse or healthcare provider, please consider going to your nearest Urgent Care or the Emergency room. As always if you feel you may be having an emergency you should call 911, or the emergency response phone number you have available to you in your country or military base.

Anxiety is a simple self-defense mechanism that is in place to help protect us from danger and situations where we might become injured. Basically, anxiety is an emotion.

This emotion is probably why to human race is still here on Earth today. Without it we would have never ran from

Saber-toothed cats, or raiding parties of Neanderthals.

## How is Anxiety Diagnosed?

Your provider will need to run a series of tests to determine whether you suffer from anxiety. Lab tests are not useful in diagnosing anxiety disorders, but in some cases might be used to evaluate whether you have electrolyte or other chemical imbalances.

Your healthcare provider will also evaluate how long you have been experiencing your anxiety, your medical and psychological history, your family history, and how the anxiety affects your daily living routine.

If your doctor can't find a medical reason for you feeling the way you are, he or she may prescribe medication for you, and/or refer you to a psychiatrist, psychologist, or other trained counselor.

It is important to note that not all psychological illnesses are covered under health insurance, so speak to your doctor to determine what other options may be available to you.

**How is Anxiety Treated?**

People who suffer from anxiety will often try more than one treatment at the same time, or at different times over the scope of their illness.

There are many medications available on the market today that can help control anxiety disorders.

Antidepressants are usually the medication of choice. Lexapro, Prozac, and Xanax are very successful in controlling the symptoms.

Psychotherapy is a type of treatment that studies the human response to anxiety as well as many other psychological conditions. The goal of psychotherapy is to find a way to help us better cope with the condition.

And Cognitive Therapy which is a way to help us to identify triggers and oncoming episodes of an anxiety attack and help us to change the behavior and thought patters that trigger the anxiety to begin with.

This book and Anxiety Control Plan is best used with the companion Anxiety Shredding Journal, by T.L. Campbell, M.S.N., R.N., available on Amazon.com.

**The Steps of Recovery**

**STEP 1: Recognition**

Recognition is the first step of recovery. You will experience certain events that made you anxious before, but you will find that they no longer bother you as they once did.

You will still experience anxiety, but on a much smaller scale that before. Remember everyone experiences stress. Stress is normal. You may experience stress over situations, but it's healthy stress, not anxiety or panic. You no longer feel you are being steam rolled by anxiety.

**STEP 2: Forgetting**

Step 2 is forgetting the anxiety. This differs from Step 1 in that when the situation arises that once caused you to duck and run for cover, you simply don't experience the uncomfortable feelings that you once had over the anxiety causing event.

**STEP 3: Living**

Step 3 is the point where you will be able to realize what affect your anxiety disorder has had on your life and start living it again.

You'll find things more interesting than ever before. You will find yourself thinking about getting out of the house, whereas before, you just wanted to crawl in bed and cover your head with the blankets.

You may catch yourself saying, "Why don't we take a trip this weekend?" or "Let invite our friends over for a bar-b-que this weekend, dear."

And finally,

**STEP 4 Resolution**

Step 4 is the greatest and most rewarding as it signifies that your commitment has paid off. Your resolution to overcoming your foe.

Anxiety will raise its ugly head again. It is only a matter of time. Resolution can take months even years to achieve fully, but you will achieve it.

Until now things have been fairly smooth, and you've gotten your life back. You are doing things that you once did before your disorder took them away, and now like a ex-lover from a bad relationship it shows up again.

What will happen then? Well, you will know how to handle it this time. You are resolute in your commitment to not take get into a self-destructive relationship with anxiety again.

You will have all the tools and techniques from this book in your head and you will be ready to unleash them at a moment's notice.

How do I know this? Because wasn't it you who Recognized the problem, learned to forget the anxiety, started living your life again, and became resolute that this is your life and you control how you want to feel? Then how can anything r anyone ever tell you any different or take that away from you again?

The day that anxiety returns for a visit will be the greatest day ever, because that's the day you'll hold up your hand and say, "**NO

**MORE ANXIETY, I'M DONE WITH YOU FOREVER!"**

**The Perception of Anxiety and Panic Attacks.**

For a good part of my like I was afraid to leave the safety of my apartment. I feared the inevitable return of a anxiety crisis that would capsize me right in front of my family.

I would have anxiety attacks waiting for the next anxiety attack to surface. Beads of sweat would appear on my forehead and drench my clothes. I would struggle to breath and expect a heart attack at any moment.

I was doomed.

My mother would tell me, "Just don't think about it." But she really had no idea what she was saying. I thought about it constantly at that point.

I would hear from my sister and friends, "Grow up and deal with it." And I would be asked, "What are you afraid of? You, big sissy."

But that's just it. I didn't know what I was afraid of, but it didn't matter. Whatever it was, had me by the throat so I was content to stay down, stay low, and hide out.

What I didn't realize then was that no matter where I was or what I did, it wasn't getting better. I was a captive to the fear of fear.

I was under attack, but I had no idea where the attack was originating.

Now I realize I wasn't a big sissy at all. What they couldn't understand was how I was being affected inside my mind. No one could understand what it was really like for me, not even my counselor.

Sure, these people were offering help in their own way, and even now when I look back on what they were saying to me, I thank them for the effort.

The longer you go through life with anxiety weighing you down, the more people will become exhausted with it and you. I lost a lot of good friends in those days, because they thought it was them I didn't want to be around.

I have helped many people over the years from 12-year-old suicidal patients, to 97-year-old widows who feel like they have nothing left in life and are unloved.

The way people perceive your anxiety disorder will be different for everyone that is why we need to help you be free of it sooner rather than later.

**You Have What It Takes to Do It.**

There is no special pill that can cure you. In fact, pills aren't the best way to beat anything.

When you take pills, you are becoming reliant on those pills to make you feel somewhat normal.

Your body compensates for the drugs you are taking in and stops making the chemical normally provided by your body and brain. The when you try to get off of the medication, there is a lag time and dependency which you go through while you wait for your body and brain to begin making those chemicals again.

Most people can't handle that and begin going through withdrawals which make the anxiety come back full force.

Now, as a registered nurse I would never ever tell you not to consider taking medications, prescribed or otherwise. But, I would tell you to consider other avenues of therapy and treatment beforehand.

There are things you are doing that are creating the anxiety in your life. That is what must be addressed and repaired so you can be free of anxiety.

You don't have to wish for a brand-new body, or some sort of bizarre electro therapy to fix your disorder. You already have what it takes to correct the problem.

Remember what I said earlier about not wanting to completely dissolve the anxiety. You can't do it. There is supposed to be some amount of stress in our lives and trying to completely do away with it is an impossible anxiety inducing pipe dream. So, the more you try to get completely stress free the more anxious you will become.

When you are stressed your body creates something called cortisol.

Cortisol is a chemical that does many things. We will keep it simple:

Let's say you're out for a walk and you happen to come across a humongous meat-eating dinosaur. I know it's sill, but let's just go with it.

The first thing that happens is you focus only on the dinosaur, and your peripheral vision dims because you can't afford to be distracted on anything else around you.

1. You become faced with a stressor, in this case, the dinosaur.

2. Your adrenal glands secrete a chemical called cortisol.

3. The cortisol prepares your body for the Fight-or-Flight reaction by flooding it with glucose, which supplies a huge boost of energy to your muscles. Peripheral vision dims, and you become extremely focused on the danger.

Here's a problem though, this instant burst of energy causes nasty side effects.

4. Cortisol narrows the arteries in your body, and epinephrine increases your heart rate, and this forces the heart to pump harder and faster. Blood pressure increases. You start sweating, trembling, and can even become nauseas. These nasty side effects are what are known as "anxiety".

5. Then you are forced to fight the beast or take flight from the meat-eating dinosaur.

6. The issue is then resolved, and the body should return to normal.

Even if the dinosaur is chasing you, you don't notice the nasty side effects because you are focused on running away and staying alive.

But in a person with an anxiety disorder this isn't what happens at all. The only reason cortisol should be released into the blood stream is to keep you safe from harm when you are in danger.

So, when you are home, safe in your bed, watching television, reading a book, or whatever, and then you begin to experience the Fight-or-Flight symptoms you notice all the nasty side effects that come along with it.

You are now having a full-blown anxiety crisis.

When this happens, it is the most frightening experience because you know it shouldn't be happening because you are safe. There is no meat-eating dinosaur to be focused on, so you experience all of the nasty side effects that cortisol brings with it.

You squirm as the pins and needles poke you all over. You struggle with catching your breath while wiping away the torrents of sweat streaming down your brow. You feel as if you are dying.

Remember, if a dinosaur was chasing you, you wouldn't even be feeling these side effects because you be too busy trying to stay alive. You don't ever want to eliminate anxiety when you are actually in danger.

So, the question is… why do you experience the Fight-or-Flight Response when you aren't actually in danger?

Well, the answer is as unbelievable as it is simple. Your brain is capable of performing trillion of processes every second. There are over 1 billion cells in the human brain. It is the most significant organ that we have and the only one capable of critical thinking, yet it can't do one simple thing.

The brain cannot tell the difference… are you ready for this? The brain cannot tell the difference from something that is REAL, and something that is a thought.

This means what ever you are thinking about, your brain will react to it as if it's real, even if it is not, and it reacts by releasing chemicals and hormones into your blood that make you feel and react in a specific way. Just like cortisol.

The normal person has roughly 65,000 thoughts a day and researches are telling us that people with anxiety disorder and panic attacks have the same thoughts almost every day, over and over, focusing on negative events.

Thinking about bad things that happened in the past, and negative things that may happen in tomorrow release cortisol into our bodies, and since your brain is unable to tell the difference from a thought that is real, or a thought that is imagined it will react to it. That is why your body is experiencing the Fight-or-Flight Response even when there is no real dinosaur.

You might think. "If I'm not thinking negative thoughts then why is it that I still have anxiety and panic attacks for no reason?" The answer is because you have been thinking these thought day after day for so long that you have a surplus of cortisol "the stress hormone" floating around in your body. This is why even when you are safe at home asleep in your bed you wake with all the nasty little Fight-or-Flight signs and symptoms.

I know how it feels. I suffered for years and years with this problem. And, like me, you've probably tried medicines alternative therapies, acupuncture, and a whole host of things that you believed would help you.

Don't let me steer you wrong, there are a lot of great things that help support you to rid yourself of anxiety, but they won't work alone.

You have been unwittingly training your brain to release cortisol "the stress hormone" for a long time and you need to break that cycle and purge the increased, unhealthy levels of cortisol from your body.

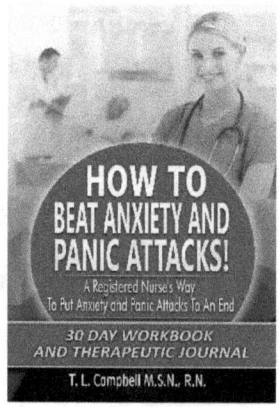

You need to retrain your brain. That is why it is so important that you don't skip any pages in this book, and why it is doubly important that you go to Amazon.com and get a copy of my *How to Beat Anxiety and Panics Attacks! 30 Day Workbook and Therapeutic Journal,* now, to help retrain your brain and say goodbye to anxiety and panic once and for all.

A major cause of anxiety is how we perceive the world we live in, but the good news is we have a big impact on how we choose to see the things which happen to us in our daily lives.

Some of the greatest minds from history suffered from anxiety disorder. It was strongly believed that Abraham Lincoln suffered from anxiety. He once said, "We live in the midst of alarms; anxiety beclouds the future; we expect some new disaster with each newspaper we read."

Others who suffered from the disorder were Emily Dickinson; one of America's most beloved literary figures, and the artist, Vincent van Gogh.

Everyone responds differently to anxiety. President Lincoln led this great country though one of the darkest times in its history, Miss Dickinson withdrew from public life, only corresponding with editors and other authors through letters, and Vincent van Gogh, suffering from various psychiatric troubles ultimately committed suicide.

They were all human beings, no different than you or I, yet they each handled the same disorder differently, just like you and me.

How you choose to respond to anxiety and panic attacks is up to you. You can control it, run from it, or let it rule over you. You are in control, and you need to know that only you control who you are, what you do, and how you react to the things that happen in our lives.

Let me offer up an example. You have a major opportunity to land the perfect job. The interview is today, so not taking a chance on being late you leave your house early, but, uh oh, there is a wreck on the highway, and the whole thing is shut down. There is no way to get off the highway and go around, so you're trapped there.

If you think, "Now I'm going to be late to the interview and they will think I'm not interested. I'll lose the job," then you are working yourself into a frenzy for no reason.

'Worry' is a useless thing. You'll start honking at the poor souls in front of you to get out of your way, but they're just as stuck as you are. Your blood pressure will skyrocket, your heart will pound, you'll start perspiring, and then the adrenals will give you a good ol' dose of cortisol. You just whipped up a good bout of Fight-or-Flight all on your own. You've made your brain believe you are in danger. Great job.

Here come all the symptoms, and since you're not really in a live threatening situation, you get to suffer through each one.

When you arrive at the interview, you look fatigued, stressed, and not focused. Your clothes are dam with sweat, your pupils are enlarged, and to make matters worse you may be nauseas, and your prospective employer is wonder what the hell is wrong with you.

There was another way, but instead you found the easiest way to handle the situation was do what you always do and let anxiety make the call.

Instead, you could have said, "This is unfortunate. I'll give the hiring manager a call and explain I'll be a few minutes late, so he or she knows I still want the job." Then you could have sat back and waited for an offramp while listening to your favorite relaxing music.

You would have avoided the entire panic attack, cortisol release and Fight-or-Flight Response. You also wouldn't have had stored excess cortisol that will be sure to be floating around in your system to wake you up in the middle of the night, for a panic attack.

At first responding correctly to a situation will take practice, and effort, but in time you will get better and better at it. In time instead of giving into anxiety you will have trained your brain to turn to logical and calmer decision-making.

# Part II: Reclaim your life

Now that you understand what anxiety is, what causes it, and how it affects you, you can use that knowledge to get control over your life again.

If you skipped any of Part I, then go back and read it. There is critical information in there that you need. You must know what anxiety is to be able to understand how to control it.

D you realize that you are on the way to curing your anxiety? That's right. You said to yourself, "I have had just about enough of this. I'm not letting this ruin my life. I took the first step and bought this book. It's helped me. Now I know what anxiety is and now I can learn to control it.

Anxiety is a multi-headed beast, so we will fight this from multiple points of attack.

**MIND.** As you have learned, what happens in your mind plays a huge part in how anxiety affects you. Remember, your brain can do so many wonderful things, but what it can't do is tell the difference between a thought and reality. If you imagine you are in danger, your mind has no other option than to believe it, otherwise your own mind would be responsible for failing to save you from danger.

Everything you need to beat anxiety and panic attacks is inside of you. You don't need to avoid places. You don't need a safe place, a security blanket, a security guard, you just need you. You need to retrain your way of thinking.

**BODY.** You've already learned what causes you to feel the way you do when you have an anxiety attack. It's that thing called cortisol coupled with the fact that you're not really in a life-threatening crisis. But what do you do when you can't stop the beast from getting in?

You'll learn techniques that will help to calm you, and you'll be able to do this without anyone's help, any medication, or running away. You have what you need already inside of you.

Controlling how your body responds to the Fight-or-Flight Response is crucial in controlling those unpleasant anxiety symptoms.

I have collected some of the best techniques that I found helped me, and they will help you to. How do I know? Because you and I are human beings. The human mind and body in all our infinite uniqueness, is biologically the identical.

If you try a technique and find it doesn't work with you go on to the next one, but don't scratch any off your list. If one doesn't work for now, it still might work for you later.

Take time to memorize these techniques, or better yet, carry this book with you wherever you go, and book mark the page. Remember overcoming your anxiety and panic attacks can be done. It will be done. You will win your life back but know that as with anything it will take commitment and practice to master these techniques.

**How Can I Control Anxiety**?

The first thing you have to do to beat anxiety and panic attacks is to commit to winning the fight.

The goal is not to make the anxiety disappear. Let me explain that another way. I have many, many parents call me asking what do when their child has a fever of 102.1. They gave ibuprofen and the fever didn't go away, it only lowered 2 or 3 degrees.

The advice I always give is that, number 1, ibuprofen won't make a fever go away completely. It only lowers the fever a few degrees at best, and number 2, fevers are beneficial to getting rid of what is making us sick? So why get rid of it completely?

It's the same with anxiety. The goal is not to be incapacitated by anxiety, panic, fear, or any other emotion. Why? Well, because stress… normal stress is a health human emotion.

What we need to understand here is that by trying to make your anxiety go away completely, the more you will try to remain completely calm, and when you fail to calm yourself completely, the more anxious you will become because you can't reach the level of peaceful tranquility you think you should be experiencing. It's a vicious cycle. Don't get caught up in it. If you do, then anxiety wins.

It's time to talk about how we are going to get to Step 1, Recognition, and to do that we have to practice. YES! I said *practice*.

Many of the steps I will give you, will be ones that you will practice. An in time, along with your commitment, you will gain control over anxiety in a few short weeks to months. Resolution will come later, but it will happen for you, just like it happened for me.

I won't lie to you. It will take effort, you may have times where you feel the anxiety and panic again, but in time you will feel it less and less, and you will be able to control the disorder and not let it control you.

As a note, this book is best used with its companion workbook, *How to Beat Anxiety, A Registered Nurse's Way to Put Anxiety and Panic Attacks to and End!* You can find it on Amazon.com.

**Self-talking.**

This technique will be very useful in stopping a problem before it starts. There is no time like the present to start learning to self-talk. It can also be helpful in the midst of an attack.

Some of the questions you may ask yourself are, *"Do I feel safe right now?"* or *"Do I do my best to focus on the positive and less on negative things?"* or *"Am I where I am supposed to be in life?"*

*"Do I feel calm and relaxed? If not, why not? What would help me feel calmer?"*

*"I will not stress out on the things I cannot change. I will accept them and make them work for me."*

*"I accept that there are things I cannot change. There are many things I cannot control, and I will learn from them."*

*"I will decide to live in the here and now and I will accept each obstacle as they come. I will overcome them one at a time."*

*"I will worry less about the future. I will grow and change and be ready for tomorrow."*

*"Negative things are not worth worrying about."*

*"I will focus on positive things and enjoy them while they are happening."*

*"If I find myself thinking about negative things, or things that make me feel anxious, I will replace them with positive thoughts."*

*"What can I do when I'm not feeling calm and relaxed? Let me name 3 activities I can do."*

**Breathing exercises.**

Controlled, slow, and deep for 5 minutes. It's one of the fastest ways to calm your anxiety.

It has been proven that breathing deeply changes the state of the mind.

Breathing slowly and deeply will help to settle the anxious mind by comforting the brain's fight or flight response.

This technique may not work for everyone right away. Sometimes it takes several attempts and even some practice to see a noticeable difference. Keep trying. Don't give up.

**Simple stretching.**

Stretching helps to decrease the stress that the body stores while sitting or laying for long periods of time.

Take a break when possible and stand up and stretch out. Stretching promotes a feeling of well-being, improves elasticity and mobility.

Start with your head, neck, shoulders, and work your fingers and toes, waist, toes, neck, and spine.

Being immobile for too long opens an opportunity for the mind to start working on stressful situations. It's okay to think about issues. Avoidance is not a good thing but having something to do while thinking of these issues will help you to cope with them better.

**Organize something small like a deck of cards.**

By placing something in order you can gain relief because it will give you a sense of mental order.

**Get away, anywhere.**

A short day-trip is a great way to get a change of scenery. A great distraction from life's everyday worries. You don't have to drive too far. A few hours in ether direction can prove fascinating and adventurous.

**Ask yourself some questions.**

*"What is the worst thing that could happen?"* Once you have an answer ask yourself,

*"What would I do, or how would I react if this happened?"* Now, you should spend some time reflecting on your answers. Visualize the way you would respond in your head. Play out the scenario in your mind.

**Take a much-needed break from working on a problem or trying to solve an issue.**

While you are taking a break from thinking about the issue, your mind will still be working on it subconsciously, and that's okay.

**Take a shower, or a bath and relax.**

When I am suffering from anxiety or stress I draw up a nice hot bath. The heated water helps to vasodilate everything and get the blood flowing. It helps the brain to reset and function better. The mind self-heals and uses the blood flow to reset your normal mood.

We all have problems and things that bother us. We are human beings and none of us have the perfect lives. Problems make us who we are. We wouldn't recognize the high points without being able to compare them to the low points. When something unexpected happens, embrace it and realize we will be better tomorrow for it.

**Do not watch the news, or the television.**

Reduce, or completely cut out the amount of television you are watching. If you must listen to the radio, choose comforting music with very little talking.

**Make a phone call to a friend or family.**

**Write a letter or email to a friend or family member. Include funny pictures of photos of family or events.**

**Finalize or complete something that you have been putting off.**

Often the things we have been avoiding are a great cause of anxiety, and we may not even realize it. By completing something you have been putting off or dreading you can mark it from your list and put it in the imaginary problem shredder.

**Try meditating.**

It's okay if you don't know how to meditate. Just find a quiet spot in your home, or a quit place in a park and relax. Think of how beautiful your surroundings are or just let your mind wander. If you find your mind going to places that trigger your anxiety, close that imaginary door and wander to another happier thought.

**Spend time with a pet.**

If you don't have a pet, consider getting one. Consider a pet that is easy to care for. Having something else in our life that distracts us from moments of anxiety is very healing. Dogs for instance are wonderful companions. They know when we are down, and they know when we are anxious. Stay away from smaller breeds as they are naturally anxious and can heighten our own anxiety. Larger dog breeds are more calm and secure.

**If a mistake you've made is bothering you, make an action plan for how you won't repeat it in the future. Write three brief bullet points.**

1. Ask yourself if you're jumping to conclusions? For example, if you're worried someone is very annoyed with you, do you know for sure this is the case or are you jumping to conclusions?

2.    Ask yourself if you're thinking the worst. For example, are you thinking that if something happened would it be the worst thing ever? Always remember and think that is something bad happens, while it might be unpleasant it won't necessarily be a disaster.

3.    Forgive yourself for not handing a situation in an ideal way, including interpersonal situations. What's the best thing you can do to move forward in a positive way now?

**The Magic Bullet**

I am about to give you the number one anxiety busting technique that will help you to overcome anxiety for good.

The *Magic Bullet* is a technique that I like to call *Reconnecting and Reasoning*. Let me explain.

Think of a time when you were nearly involved in a car accident. Now think of the feelings that it caused you at that moment. Your heart raced as adrenaline raced through your system. Your breath quickened, your legs may have gone numb or began tingling. Your chest tightened I expectation of what was about to happen. That's because your brain sensed danger and became afraid.

When you are having an anxiety crisis, or you wake up in the middle of a panic attack your brain is sensing danger and has become afraid.

Most people immediately get up out of bed and began pacing or some other avoidance type of behavior. Your brain will sense this as confirmation as what it is doing by being fearful and being afraid is justified and that you are MOVING AWAY from danger.

This sets up a vicious cycle where your brain, for what ever reason becomes afraid and you move away from an unreal, unknown danger. Therefore, your brain will get to the point where it takes less and less for anything to trigger that anxiety/panic mode with the attempt to keep you safe. It will begin to over react to every stressor you come across, real or imagined it will make no difference.

So, what we need to do is retrain your brain. And yes, you can do it. You are no different than anyone else with anxiety disorder.

First, we need to reconnect out thoughts, so our brain can acquire reasoning.

When you are deep into an anxiety or panic attack what you must do is think of a thought that excites you in a positive way.

Think of something good, like a day out with a friend, an upcoming event, seeing your grandkids this weekend, etc. and imagine how good it makes you feel to think of the prospect of doing that thing.

We need to focus on this positive thought and hold onto it. Think of it intensely. Imagine seeing your grandchildren, kissing and hugging them, imagine the conversation you will have with your friend and what you will do together, imagine the great kiss you and your date will share.

Do not let go of that thought. If you feel yourself thinking of anything else refocus on the positive thought again.

Your brain will begin reasoning that your heart must be pounding, not from fear, but from positively generated excitement. The fearfulness that your brain was feeling will dissolve and be replaced by positive feeling, and more pleasurable sensations.

Each and every time you have an anxiety or panic attack, from that point on, you must go back to your *prechosen* positive thought and focus on it again.

In time your brain will begin to react less and less to an unreasonable fear and begin reasoning that it only needs to react to positive and pleasurable stimuli.

As always, remember, your goal is not to try to completely get rid of stress, because stress is healthy when we deal with it appropriately, and we

are in control.

# Part III: Putting it all together

We've discussed the cause of your anxiety and panic attack and we've covered various techniques to correct them before and during the attack.

It's time for you to demonstrate what you have learned. There are two ways to do just that.

When I was a little child my step-father would take me swimming at the apartment complex's pool. The problem was I didn't know how to swim, and I was deathly afraid of drowning.

His way of teaching was for me to enter into the deep end and face my fear of drowning head on. Open myself to my fears and take them on, instead of cowering from them. Although I didn't see it then, what he was trying to do is have me face the fear of the fear.

Even though I felt the fear taking a lose grip on my throat I didn't run away from it, because running away would have made the anxiety worse. The fear would have been back and stronger than ever before the next time I came to the swimming pool.

If you are avoiding the grocery store, the movie theater, a restaurant, or a family event, then you are telling yourself that these places and events are a threat to you. You give power to fear and open a door for anxiety to walk through as much as it pleases.

To overcome the fear and deliver a mortal wound to anxiety you must face your fear head on.

I remember filling my lungs with life giving air, pinching my nose, and jumping into the deep in. Of course, I floundered to the side of the pool like a drunken octopus, but I faced the fear on my own. The pool was no longer a scary or dangerous place for me. From that point onward, I lived at the pool during Summer vacation.

The other way to demonstrate what you have learned is don't plan ahead. This means if you know you are going to be doing something or going somewhere that causes you to be anxious or panic, don't think about it.

If you plan try to plan out the event that usually causes your anxiety, your mind will constantly work on you and try to stop you from living your life and doing what you want to do.

Your mind isn't doing this to you because it hates you. It's doing it because it loves you, it wants to keep you free from harm, because without you there is no mind. If something happens to you then it happens to your mind too. It's self-preservation to the extreme.

If you experience your anxiety when get to the place that usually triggers it or the event that brings it on, then remember your techniques and put them into action.

**When anxiety comes back**

What should you do if anxiety or panic attacks return?

The problem is that they may return and in many cases they will return.

A friend recently contacted me who I haven't heard from in years. When I asked him how he was doing, he told that he had been doing fine and then all of the sudden the anxiety began to get worse for him again.

Anxiety is shift character and will constantly look for a wat to cause chaos in your life.

After a lengthy chat we had come up with a new plan. All he needed was a little tune-up. He had been using the same techniques that worked for him initially without trying to use any other techniques.

We simply worked in some new techniques and I got him to talk with me about any new stressors in his life. After a few weeks he called me again telling me things were back on track for him. The important thing was he realized the symptoms early and was able to react and adapt.

When anxiety comes back into your life don't look at that as a failure. It isn't a failure at all, it's an opportunity for you to rise above it and be victorious over the disorder that has plagued your life for so long.

I highly encourage you to go to amazon.com and pic up a copy of

I strongly encourage you to go to Amazon.com and get a copy of my *How to Beat Anxiety! 30 Day Workbook and Therapeutic Journal,* now, to help retrain your brain and say goodbye to anxiety and panic once and for all.

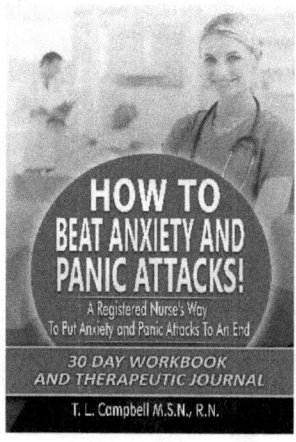

This 30-Day Workbook is instrumental in helping you develop a routine and retrain your brain. It will offer you a way to express yourself in a therapeutic way and find a pathway to a cure.

Thank you for reading this book. I hope and trust that you are on your way to defeating the beast we call anxiety. I pray that your sleep with be free from panic attacks, and I truly believe you have taken the most important first step in freeing yourself from the chains of anxiety disorder.

If you enjoyed this book, please give it a great rating on Amazon.com right now. Without your rating and positive review, we can't hope to get this material to others who

are suffering just like you.


Thank you again,

Trace Campbell, M.S.N., R.N.


If you would like to reach the author,

please write to TraceCampbell@hotmail.com

www.ingramcontent.com/pod-product-compliance
Lightning Source LLC
Chambersburg PA
CBHW080842220526
45467CB00008B/2352